Kids and Alcohol, the Deadliest Drug

Also by Stanley L. Englebardt

Jobs in Health Care
Careers in Data Processing

Kids and Alcohol, the Deadliest Drug

Stanley L. Englebardt

Lothrop, Lee & Shepard Company
A Division of William Morrow & Company, Inc.

New York

1 2 3 4 5   79 78 77 76 75
Library of Congress Cataloging in Publication Data
Englebardt, Stanley L
    Kids and alcohol, the deadliest drug.
    Bibliography: p.
    Includes index.
    SUMMARY: An introduction to alcohol—what it is, how it affects the body, why some people become problem drinkers, and how to recognize, prevent and treat alcoholism.
    1. Alcohol and youth—United States—Juvenile literature. 2. Alcoholism—Juvenile literature. 3. Alcohol—Physiological effect—Juvenile literature [1. Alcohol. 2. Alcoholism] I. Title.
HV5066.E54   362.2′92′0973   75-20327
ISBN 0-688-41717-5
ISBN 0-688-51717-X lib. bdg.

Acknowledgments

Many people and events are involved in the genesis of a book. It would be impossible to remember or acknowledge all of the individuals who provided ideas, insights, and information for *Kids and Alcohol, the Deadliest Drug*. Some of the material used in this book was picked up casually at professional symposiums and at informal dinner parties; some of it came from daily perusal of journals, magazines, and newspapers; some of it was the result of research on the subject of alcoholism. Nevertheless, there are sources which stand out in my memory—and I would like to offer these people a particular thanks.

Among the first to bring my attention to the growing problem of alcohol abuse among young people was Dr. Paul Kaunitz, a practicing psychiatrist and Professor of Psychiatry at Yale University Medical School. Dr. Kaunitz, who had been active in the area of teenage alcoholism long before it became of concern to many of his colleagues, sought me out at a social function to tell me why he thought the subject deserved national attention.

Shortly after Dr. Kaunitz planted the seed, Dr. Harold Rockaway, chief of psychiatry at St. Joseph's Hospital in Houston, Texas, nurtured it with some observations of his own. Dr. Rockaway, who has spent most of his medical career working with hard-core adult alcoholics, told me that for the first time he was beginning to see numbers of extremely ill teenage alcoholics. "I'm concerned," he said, "and I think it's about time the public realized what's going on with their children."

In addition, I owe a debt of gratitude to the personnel of the National Institute on Alcohol Abuse and Alcoholism who patiently answered all my questions and provided literally reams of material about alcohol use and abuse in the United States. Dr. Morris E. Chafetz, director of the National Institute, and the many scientists who work with him are to be commended for their efforts on behalf of the people of the United States.

Finally, I must mention the important contributions made by my wife and children. They listened to every word of my copy, made valuable suggestions, and provided the proper environment for getting the book done. Moreover, my son Lee, a college student, and my daughter Lynn, a high school student, gave me the benefit of their observations of drinking among their peers.

S.L.E.

Contents

1 • Alcohol, the Drug of Choice Among Young People • 9

A Growing Problem of Abuse
Part of a National Problem
The Many Hazards of Drinking
The Need to Understand Alcohol and Alcoholism

2 • What It Is, and How It Affects Your Body • 16

The Chemistry of Alcoholic Beverages
How Alcohol Makes You "Drunk"
Why Some People Hold Their Liquor Better Than Others

3 • What Drinking Can Do to Your Health • 24

Short-term Effects of Alcohol
Long-term Effects of Alcohol
Related Problems

4 • How and Why Some People Become "Problem Drinkers" • 29

The Difference Between "Problem Drinkers" and "Alcoholics"
Profile of the Problem Drinker
Signs of the True Alcoholic
The Last Stages

5 • Are You a Candidate for Alcoholism? • 37

Common Factors
Research into the Causes of Alcoholism
A Formula for Avoiding Alcoholism

6 • How to Recognize, Prevent, and Treat Alcoholism • 45

The Three Stages of Treatment
Counseling
Psychotherapy
Involving the Entire Family
Behavior and Aversion Therapy
Alcoholics Anonymous
Helping Families of Alcoholics
Where to Go for Help

7 • Some Questions and Answers About Alcohol • 55

References • 60

Index • 62

1 Alcohol, the Drug of Choice Among Young People

Nobody has to tell you that kids have discovered a new drug. The name of this "new" substance: alcohol. It's inexpensive, easy to obtain and, essentially, legal. You can find it today on virtually all college campuses, in most junior and senior high schools, and in many elementary schools. According to one government survey, the use of alcohol by young people during the past four years has almost doubled. More frightening, the number of kids who are now *abusing* this drug—that is, drinking to the point where it causes some harm to their body or mind—is increasing at an alarming rate.

All the signs and surveys show that a major switch in drug choice has taken place. In 1972, when the newspapers, magazines, and broadcast media were talking mainly about the widespread abuse of drugs such as heroin, LSD, marijuana, a federal study showed that more than twice as many young people were drinking liquor as were smoking "pot". In fact, according to the government statistics, the *drug of choice* among the vast majority of pre-teens and teen-agers was alcohol.

Many adults found these figures hard to believe. After all, they didn't see any junior high school kids lined up at bars, staggering down the street, or flopping on skid row. That was the kind of alcohol abuse they expected only from other adults. Young people, they thought, had another kind of poison.

But then, in 1974, the U.S. Department of Health, Education and Welfare organized the largest study ever run on the use of alcohol by young people. Trained researchers were sent to junior and senior high schools all across the country to find out just what was really going on. They assured the kids they were interviewing that they were interested only in statistics, and nobody would get in trouble for telling the truth. Not only did these teenagers confirm the earlier findings, but they added some new dimensions to the alcohol use picture. Here, for example, are some of the things that the researchers found out about alcohol use and abuse by young people in the United States today:

• Kids in grades seven through twelve are using alcohol today more often than at any other time in history.

• Among seventh graders, who average about twelve years of age, some 63 percent of the boys and 54 percent of the girls told the researchers that they'd used alcohol at least once.

• Among the junior and senior high kids they spoke to, the number who admitted to having tried alcohol at least once increased with each grade unit. When the researchers talked to high school seniors, about 93 percent of the boys and 87 percent of the girls admitted they had had one or more drinks at some time in their life.

A Growing Problem of Abuse

I'm sure that very few young people are surprised by these figures. As a matter of fact, many of the junior and senior high kids who participated in the study said they'd taken their first drink at a family party, sipping it right in front of their parents and family friends. "There's no big deal about a kid having a drink," says a junior high student. "After all, one drink doesn't make an alcoholic any more than one robin makes a spring."

But the number of young people who have tried alcohol at least once is really only the visible tip of a very large iceberg. What you don't see—and what worries health authorities—is the growing number of pre-teens and teenagers who are now using alcohol regularly as a means of blotting out reality. For example, the HEW study showed that nearly one out of every four junior and senior high kids got "high" or "bombed" at least four times a year, and one out of every seven male high school seniors got drunk at least once a week.

Does getting drunk a few times a year mean that someone is an alcoholic? Not necessarily—but it may mean that they already have a drinking problem. Consider some of the other signs which reveal just how far alcohol abuse has gone in recent years:

• In the last ten years, arrests of girls eighteen and younger for what the law calls "public drunkenness" has more than tripled, while arrests of boys in the same age group has more than doubled. Arrests for public drunkenness usually mean that the individuals involved were causing enough of a disturbance to attract the attention of the police.

• Where no Alcoholics Anonymous groups for children and teenagers existed before 1970, now there are six such chapters in the New York City area alone and four in Los Angeles. Other teenage chapters are springing up all over the country. Moreover, where it used to be extremely rare to find a teenager or pre-teen in an AA meeting, now many chapters have a sizeable teenage membership.

• Where drug treatment centers such as Synanon and Phoenix

House rarely, if ever, saw an alcoholic youngster five years ago, now they report that from 10 to 50 percent of their membership are under-seventeen-year-old problem drinkers.

• Where drinking was virtually unheard of among elementary school students in 1970, now problem drinkers are being found at every grade level. A recent study of over 9,500 junior and senior high students by three Hunter College professors revealed that 40 percent of the kids had started using beer or wine well before their seventh grade. Some elementary school teachers have reported finding either drunken or severely hung-over children as early as kindergarten and the first grade.

Part of a National Problem

"Okay," says a Seattle, Washington, high school junior, "so some kids do drink too much. But it seems to me that adults use and abuse alcohol a lot more than any teenager I know."

The Seattle student is absolutely correct. According to the latest available figures, alcohol consumption among adults has gone up a whopping 26 percent in the last ten years. In 1974, in fact, enough beer, wine, and hard liquor was sold in the United States to provide every man and woman over the age of twenty-one with 2.6 gallons of straight alcohol.

"If it's adults who do most of the heavy drinking, then why single out young people for following their example?" asks the same youngster.

Good question—and there are at least two solid reasons why this book is directed to young people.

First, because today's young problem drinkers are almost certain to become tomorrow's adult alcoholics. Alcoholism is a serious disease which can cause almost unbelievable pain and suffering. Recent studies have shown that the earlier a child starts drinking, the more liable he or she is to become an alcoholic later in life. Therefore, by learning about alcohol *before* it becomes a problem, we may be able to prevent some of this future misery.

Second, because young people who have not yet attained their full physical and intellectual growth are particularly susceptible to the effects of alcohol. Those effects can range from liver disease and intestinal irritation to impaired thinking processes. No matter what they are, though, there's evidence that the problem starts earlier and progresses faster in most young people than it does in adults. Thus, by preventing alcohol abuse now, we may be able to save many pre-teen and teenage drinkers from a variety of near-future physical and emotional problems.

The Many Hazards of Drinking

Whether or not you use alcoholic beverages may seem like a purely personal decision. What you have to learn, though, is that alcohol is an insidious drug and many of its most devastating effects are beyond your control. More important, those effects can cause suffering, disability, and death to innocent bystanders just as frequently as they cause destruction to the drinker. Consider:

• Out of the 95 million Americans who drink alcoholic beverages, at least 9 million are "hooked" on the drug. They cannot control their drinking habit and will do almost anything to satisfy their daily alcohol needs. As a result, they cause harm not only to themselves, but to all the people around them who are forced to live with and take care of the drinker's problem.

• Alcohol is, in one way or another, responsible for taking more than 85,000 lives each year. More than half of the 50,000 deaths of Americans in highway accidents each year, for example, are the direct result of drinking. This doesn't mean that all the victims were drunk at the time of the accident. In many cases they were simply innocent passengers in automobiles smashed by drunken drivers.

The same is true of many of the murders which are committed each year. Police records show that in at least half of all homicides the killer was under the influence of alcohol at the time of the act. Maybe this is why so many murderers say, "I didn't know what I was doing."

Drinking causes an untold amount of family suffering each year. In one quarter of all suicides, for example, alcohol is a factor; and more than seven times as many marriages end in legal separation or divorce when one or both of the partners has a drinking problem.

Alcoholism costs the nation about fifteen billion dollars a year. Some of the expense comes from the need for public facilities to treat alcoholics; some of it is caused by increased welfare payments to the families of alcoholics; and much of it comes from lost wages and lessened productivity of drinkers who just cannot make it to their jobs. In recent years some of this annual expense has been accounted for by young people who, because of their drinking problem, fail to attend or drop out from school.

The Need To Understand Alcohol and Alcoholism

Curiosity or a desire to appear more grown-up may be the reason why most young people take their first drink of an alcoholic beverage. Once they start, few consciously decide to continue to the point where they are abusing the substance. Nevertheless, many junior and senior high school kids today are either already hooked on alcohol or are on the brink of a real drinking problem.

"The misuse of alcohol represents a major health problem in the United States," says Dr. Morris E. Chafetz, Director of the National Institute on Alcohol Abuse and Alcoholism. "So far, we have been unable to find any simple remedy for this problem through legal or moral pressures. If we are to prevent the abuse of alcohol, we will have to understand the people who misuse it, their reasons, and the ways in which it affects them. Similarly, we need to understand the factors that encourage others to drink responsibly and moderately."

In a large sense, Dr. Chafetz's statement is what this book is all about. There is no longer any doubt that alcohol is the drug of choice among young people in the United States. It's time we learned something about alcohol and alcoholism.

2
What It Is, and How It Affects Your Body

Alcohol has had a long and colorful history. Hundreds of thousands of years ago—possibly as long as two hundred million years ago, say some experts—our prehistoric ancestors discovered that a strange thing happened when honey, fruits, berries, cereals and other plant materials were mixed with water and left in the warmth of the sun. After a while, the fruity liquid turned into a beverage with magical powers. It could dull pain, brighten the spirits, even aid communion with the gods. Little wonder, then, that this strange drink soon became a significant part of most religious or ritualistic ceremonies.

As for documented evidence of alcohol's early beginnings, we have only to look at the earliest records of the ancient Egyptians, Hebrews, Greeks, and Romans. Their writings contain countless references to alcoholic substances. Beer and wine, for example, were used by those people for medicine, as well as to produce relaxation, tranquillity, and a general feeling of comfort. When Christianity came along, alcoholic substances quickly became a part of its religious ritual.

Yet, from the very beginning, alcohol proved to be a two-faced companion. On the one hand, it did produce the peace and good feelings described so glowingly by the ancient Greeks and Romans. On the other, there were also many mentions in early literature of its harmful effects. Said the early eighteenth-century Frenchman François de Salignac de La Mothe-Fénelon, "Some of the most dreadful mischiefs that afflict mankind proceed from wine; it is the cause of disease, quarrels, sedition, idleness, aversion to labor, and every species of domestic disorder."

What is this substance which creates such strong yet opposite reactions? To understand how and why alcohol affects the body and mind in such different ways, let's first learn something about the substance.

The Chemistry of Alcoholic Beverages

Look into the window of a liquor store and you can see many different types of alcoholic beverages, as well as scores of different brands. For our purposes, we can break them down into five basic kinds of alcoholic drinks which are used socially, religiously and, sometimes, in clinical medicine. They are: beers, table wines, dessert or cocktail wines, liqueurs or cordials, and distilled spirits which are often called "hard" liquor.

In a window of a store, or lined up behind a bar, these various beverages look very different. In fact, their taste, color, and aroma can vary greatly, from the frothy, thick and bitter-tasting brew of an imported European beer to the crystal-clear, colorless and sharp taste of an American gin. Nevertheless, the main ingredient or constituent of all these beverages is a substance called ethyl alcohol. And it is the alcohol that produces intoxication and has an influence on the brain and other body organs.

Essentially, the alcohol present in all intoxicating beverages is a

What It Is, and How It Affects Your Body • 17

colorless, flammable liquid which is created by a natural process called fermentation. There are many ways in which fermentation can be set up, started, and controlled. Generally, though, it happens only when tiny colonies of bacteria are either already present in or added to a sugary liquid. Given the proper time, temperature, and environment, the sugar and bacteria will react chemically to produce a third substance which we call alcohol.

Why then do alcoholic beverages differ so much in their appearance, taste, and aroma? The difference has to do with the materials used in the process. Here, for example, is how some popular beverages are made:

• Although modern beers differ widely in their taste and appearance, all are started with a substance called brewers' wort. This is a "mash" of crushed barley malt mixed with hot water. Gradually the soluble substances in this mash are dissolved, and the starch in the mix is converted into sugar. Then, after several more steps to remove the sugary liquid from the undissolved grains, bacteria are added in the form of yeast. Final result: one of the many types of beers or ales which are so widely consumed today.

• Wine making is as old as beer making, and the techniques involved are about equally complicated. The starting ingredient in this case is grapes, which are picked at the height of their growing season, crushed and strained, and allowed to stand over a period of time. Although bacteria are deliberately added to some wines, most depend for their fermentation on a natural yeast which settles on the grape skins during the growing season. The variations in wine which are so loudly extolled by some connoisseurs come from such factors as the type of grape, the soil of the vineyard, the climate, the harvesting methods, and the time and conditions of storage.

• Distilled spirits, or "hard" liquors, come from fruits, cereals, potatoes, molasses, and many other sources of cheap, fermentable sugar. The most popular types of distilled liquor include the whiskies

—scotch, made primarily from malted barley and corn; bourbon, made from corn, rye, and malted barley; and rye, made from rye and malted barley—rum, made from sugar cane or molasses; gin, made from a variety of grains flavored by juniper berries; and vodka, which used to be made from potato starch but now is made from cereal grains or even from such diverse products as molasses or wood pulp.

What makes these whiskies and similar drinks so much more potent than, say, the beers or wines? The answer has to do with the process of distillation which, in effect, removes the solid or undissolved particles in the liquor and concentrates the alcohol. This is essentially the same technique which is used to make distilled (pure) water.

As for the potency or strength of the various alcoholic beverages, this depends on the amount of alcohol in the substance and the size of the serving. Most American beers contain about 4 percent alcohol. Table wines, such as Chablis or Bordeaux, range from 8 to 12 percent alcohol. And distilled spirits, such as scotch or rye whisky, have from 40 percent (80 proof) to 50 percent (100 proof) alcohol. Therefore a 12-ounce can of beer, a 4-ounce glass of wine, or a one-ounce jigger of 100 proof whisky will all have about the same amount of alcohol and, under similar drinking conditions, will produce about the same amount of intoxication.

How Alcohol Makes You "Drunk"

By strict definition, alcohol is a food. Although it has no nutritional value—no vitamins, no minerals, no protein—it does contain a lot of calories. Considering that it is made from sugar, this should come as no surprise. In fact, alcoholic drinks are one of the first things that should be eliminated by people who are overweight.

What concerns us here, though, is not alcohol's role in the diet, but how it acts as a drug. Unlike most other foods which we swallow, alcohol does not have to be digested. Instead, it passes directly through the walls of the stomach and small intestine where it is absorbed immediately into the bloodstream. The blood, in turn, carries it rapidly to the brain where its primary effect is on the central nervous system.

Any teenager who has tried even one drink knows that its effects can be felt within a matter of minutes. Although alcohol is a depressant, at first it acts like a stimulant, helping the drinker to become more lively and less inhibited. This is because the initial effect of the alcohol is on the upper or "newer" part of the brain where learned behavior patterns, such as self-control, are stored. Thus, particularly if the drink is taken slowly and with food, there is a tendency to "loosen up" evidenced by louder talk, easier laughter, and more willingness to socialize.

It should be noted, however, that not everyone reacts this way. For some people who may have emotional problems which are usually kept under control by the upper part of the brain, the first drink or two may produce aggressive behavior or even deep sadness.

As high blood-alcohol levels are reached through continued drinking, more and more brain cells are influenced by the alcohol. As with any other drug, alcohol's physical or physiological effects depend upon its concentration in body tissues. In this case, the higher amounts or concentrations of alcohol in the blood slow down brain cell activity to the point where memory, muscular coordination, and balance are impaired. At this stage the drinker is obviously intoxicated, with eyes glassy and empty-looking, speech thick and slurred, memory faulty and forgetful, and walk rolling or staggering.

What happens if such an individual continues to drink? In effect, the depressant action of the drug works its way deeper and deeper into the brain. Eventually enough of the brain's vital cells will be affected to produce dizziness, nausea, confusion, disorientation, stupor, anesthesia, coma and, in some cases, even death.

Why Some People Hold Their Liquor Better Than Others

You've probably heard some kids boast that they have "a hollow leg" or can "drink like a fish." Is it true that some people can hold their liquor better than others? Although sooner or later alcohol will catch up with every drinker, there are five factors that can influence how fast a person becomes drunk:

• How they drink alcoholic beverages. It has been demonstrated many times that the more rapidly a given drink is consumed, the more likely it is that the drinker will wind up intoxicated. It takes the body about one hour to metabolize, or burn up, a half ounce of alcohol. If someone exceeds this half-ounce-per-hour speed limit by gulping one or more drinks quickly, then the blood-alcohol concentration will build up rapidly to the point where it influences brain cells. Thus, the slow sipper will almost always remain in control of his mind and body longer than the rapid gulper.

• The body weight. As a rule, pre-teens and teenagers will get intoxicated faster from a given amount of alcohol than will adults. The reason for this, in most cases, is body weight. Measurements have shown that the blood-alcohol level reached in a 180-pound man drinking four ounces of distilled spirits will be substantially lower than the amount found in a 120-pound teenager drinking the same quantity in the same period of time.

• The presence of food in the stomach. One old wives' tale about alcohol happens to be true: food does influence the speed and degree of intoxication. Drinking on an empty stomach is never a good idea, because without some food present to act as a sponge, all the alcohol in the drink will race right through and into the bloodstream. If a person drinks while eating a substantial meal, on the other hand, the rate of absorption may be retarded enough to lower the blood-alcohol concentration by as much as fifty percent.

• What you drink. While all alcoholic beverages contain some amount of intoxicating substance, the percentage varies considerably from drink to drink. As we've seen, beers and wines contain much less alcohol per ounce than distilled spirits. Moreover, both beer and wine contain a fair amount of nonalcoholic substances, called congeners, which help to slow down the alcohol absorption process.

Then, too, if a drink is diluted with water or fruit juice the absorption rate will be reduced. Bear in mind, though, that diluting with carbonated mixers, such as ginger ale or club soda, will have an opposite effect and may actually *increase* the rate of absorption.

• Individual tolerance. No two people react to alcohol in exactly the same way. Some people have what doctors call the "dumping syndrome," which means that their stomach empties more rapidly than usual, and thus the alcohol gets into their bloodstream and affects their brain cells that much sooner. Then again, such things as anger, fear, stress and even recent illness can cause the stomach to empty more quickly than usual, causing faster intoxication.

What you *think* should happen can also influence the way you react to alcohol. Pre-teens sneaking a can of beer have been known to get "drunk" even though their blood-alcohol concentration has barely reached a point where it influences brain cells. Why? "Because that's the way they think they should act," says a psychologist.

The length of time people have been using alcohol, too, can influence how fast they get drunk. Chronic drinkers, it has been observed, develop a tolerance to liquor which causes them to drink more and more in order to get drunk. Young drinkers, on the other hand, may get high very quickly because their body is not yet accustomed to alcohol.

As for ways of sobering up, you can forget all the stories you've heard about sure-fire methods. As a general rule, it will take as many hours as the number of drinks consumed to recover from the effects of alcohol. And no amount of black coffee, cold showers, breathing pure oxygen or any other process can change this formula.

Finally, we come to the hangover—that morning-after misery of throbbing headache, aching muscles, queasy stomach, and stretched-tight nerves. The hangover is a common and universally unpleasant result of drinking too much. Although the exact physical mechanism of the hangover is still unknown to medical science, there is some evidence that it may be caused by a vitamin deficiency, dehydration, or the fusel oils which are present in many alcoholic beverages. Whatever the reason for it, the only way to relieve the symptoms is with aspirin, bed rest, and solid food as soon as possible.

While this may sound somewhat like a formula for healthy and happy drinking, it is intended only to help separate fact from fiction about alcohol. This book recognizes that alcoholic substances are readily available, legal in most states for people over eighteen, and a familiar aspect of daily life. While abstinence from alcohol is the only sure way of avoiding the perils of abuse, it is a fact that many pre-teens and teenagers have already experimented with beer, wine, or whiskey and may even be using these substances more or less regularly. For this reason, a little bit of knowledge can go a long way— maybe far enough to keep you from getting hooked.

3 What Drinking Can Do to Your Health

It happened in my home town just a few days before Christmas. Four high school students attended a party where they drank several beers. When it came time to leave, the host suggested that the sixteen-year-old driver might not be in condition to handle his car.

"No way," said the teenager. "I can hold my liquor and I know what I'm doing."

Looking at him, you could only agree. He was clear-eyed, steady on his feet and seemingly in complete control. Certainly not what you'd call drunk.

A few minutes later, though, he decided to show the three other sixteen-year-olds in the car how well the vehicle could hold the winding country road. He floored the accelerator and the speedometer needle climbed steadily to 60 miles per hour.

Suddenly the steering wheel seemed to pull right out of his hands. The car veered left, across the center line and into the path of an oncoming sedan.

The cars met almost head-on. The occupants of the other vehicle, a husband and wife returning from a holiday shopping excursion, were killed instantly. The teenage driver bled to death while police tried desperately to free him from the twisted metal. The sixteen-year-old girl beside him died several hours later, of head injuries, in

KIDS AND ALCOHOL, THE DEADLIEST DRUG

a local hospital. Miraculously, the two kids in the back seat escaped without a scratch—although the emotional scars of the accident will be with them for a lifetime.

Most people—kids and adults—who have had a drink or two are convinced that they can handle their car better than when they're stone-cold sober. But this is just *not true!* Dozens of scientific studies have shown beyond doubt that even a small concentration of alcohol in the bloodstream will change your judgment and physical reactions. And when you are at the controls of potentially dangerous machinery such as an automobile, these subtle changes can make you a threat to yourself and others.

Short-term Effects of Alcohol

Although drinkers differ from one another in their susceptibility to alcohol, almost all will experience some measurable change in their ability to perform motor tests after having had only a small amount of liquor. One series of studies conducted with college-age student volunteers, for example, showed that as little as 0.10 percent concentration of alcohol in the blood will slow both hand and foot reaction speed by a fraction of a second. This may not sound like much, but it is enough to make the difference between avoiding an obstacle by stopping in time or hitting it head-on. Thus, the teenager who drives after drinking only one or two beers just cannot perform as well as he or she might while alcohol-free.

Another vital physical reaction that can be changed by just a few drinks is your resistance to glare. Researchers have discovered that drinking lengthens the amount of time it takes for the eyes to readjust after being exposed to the glare of oncoming headlights. This period may be long enough to make the driver temporarily blind after going past a stream of particularly bright headlights.

Many so-called drunk-driver accidents take place at night because the driver just cannot see the road or any obstacles ahead.

Individuals who have had a few drinks tend to underestimate speed and distance. In one study, a group of drivers were tested before and after having about three ounces of liquor. In over seventy percent of the cases, their average driving speed on a driving simulater went up; and in over ninety percent of the cases they underestimated the amount of distance they'd covered. These findings suggest that alcohol tends to alter perception by making time appear to pass more slowly.

Moderate amounts of alcohol will have a pronounced effect on your emotions. Studies have shown that drinking tends to increase the likelihood of an individual's taking risks simply because he or she has decreased feelings of fear. Another way of saying this is that drinking tends to give you "false courage" in situations where you might otherwise back away or avoid contact. This has been demonstrated in a laboratory with animals who, after being given alcohol, overcame their fear of electric shock in retrieving food. Among people, this same pattern is seen in the inclination to take on bigger and stronger people in fights or to drive at speeds which sober thinking would show to be much too fast for the road or the conditions.

Moderate drinking may also reduce the sense of smell and taste. One of the first symptoms of deep intoxication is a feeling of numbness in the tongue, lips, gums and roof of the mouth. Before local anesthesia was discovered, in fact, many dentists used liquor to deaden the pain of a tooth extraction.

Long-term Effects of Alcohol

It has never been demonstrated clearly that social drinking—that is, taking alcohol in moderation, under control and within the limits of the law—causes any harm to body organs. A small amount of alcohol sipped slowly is metabolized or burned up by the body just like any other sugar-based food. It is only when the drinking habit increases and continues over a long period of time that any medical problems occur.

The range of diseases which can and do develop in heavy drinkers is staggering. One of the most obvious effects of long-term drinking is muscle disease and tremors. Called alcoholic myopathy, it usually starts as severe muscle cramps in the arms and legs, progresses after a while to acute muscle pain, swelling and weakness, and reaches its height in severe twitching, tremor, and sometimes kidney failure. In the last stage, the disease causes almost 100 percent disability, making the alcoholic useless for almost any activity but drinking. Most of these victims die many years before their normal life expectancy.

Another common result of chronic drinking is heart disease. Recent research shows that alcohol has a direct effect on the heart muscle. Under the influence of heavy drinking, your heart may not pump as hard as it should. And this, in turn, can lead to an oxygen deficiency which may result in a fatal heart attack.

Perhaps the most widespread result of heavy drinking, and one that is being found with increasing frequency among young alcoholics these days, is a liver disease called cirrhosis. The liver is the body organ most significantly involved with the processing or metabolism of alcohol, as well as other foods. For this reason, cirrhosis of the liver, which is characterized by progressive destruction of the liver's cells, occurs about six times more often among heavy drinkers than it does among non- or social drinkers. Many pre-teen and teen-age problem drinkers are first discovered when they are brought in to a doctor or a hospital suffering from the early signs of liver cirrhosis.

Alcohol is responsible for a wide range of stomach and gastrointestinal ailments. This is particularly true in young drinkers whose intestinal tissues are ultrasensitive to the irritating effects of liquor. At first this irritation is seen in the form of frequent vomiting, diarrhea, and indigeston. Later, if the drinking habit continues, the individual may develop ulcers, gastritis, and inflammation of the pancreas. If alcohol consumption continues after that, some doctors believe that the final result may be cancer of the stomach or related organs.

Related Problems

Very heavy drinkers often have a lowered resistance to pneumonia and other infectious diseases. The reason for this has to do with a by-product of drinking, rather than with the alcohol itself. Chronic drinkers characteristically get most of their calories from liquor. Without a proper diet, sooner or later their body's defenses against bacteria and viruses will become weakened. As a result, the problem drinker is unable to fight off many of the infections which a healthier person would be able to resist.

It is obvious that drinking, in any quantity, carries some very real risks. While moderate or social drinking produces no body harm, it does make the individual more prone to accident—particularly if he slides behind the wheel of a car. For chronic or long-term heavy drinkers, the chances of coming down with a serious disease are very good.

4 How and Why Some People Become "Problem Drinkers"

Most of us think of an alcoholic in terms of the skid row bum, unshaven and disheveled, sprawled in a doorway with a wine bottle in his hand.

You must have seen such unfortunate individuals at one time or another. They can be found in virtually every city and town of the United States. Yet, in fact, only three to five percent of all Americans who are problem drinkers actually fit this description.

Where are the other 95 percent?

They are all around us, seemingly carrying on a normal life. They are male and female, black and white, businessmen and laborers, housewives and secretaries, honor students and dropouts, family people and loners. It has been estimated that more than 70 percent of the nation's alcoholics reside in respectable neighborhoods, live with their family, attend church, and perform their household, business or school duties at a more or less effective level. Nevertheless, these people are just as hooked on alcohol as their skid row counterparts. More significantly, they account for most of the physical, mental, social, and emotional cost associated with alcoholism.

The Difference Between "Problem Drinkers" and "Alcoholics"

You may have noticed that sometimes in this book we talk about "alcoholics" and at other times use the phrase "problem drinkers." What is the difference?

Physicians who work in the field of alcoholism usually make a distinction between individuals who have a drinking problem and those who are true alcoholics. This difference, however, is really just a matter of degree. And it is only in the most extreme cases of alcoholism that we can make a firm diagnosis.

To provide a definition of an alcoholic, for example, we have only to go back to that picture of the skid row bum. You don't have to be a doctor or other professional in the field of alcoholism to know that anyone who allows himself to get into this condition must be very sick. The individual who sinks as low as skid row has lost all concern about his appearance, pride, health, family, and future. He exists, in effect, only for the next drink and, in most cases, will do almost anything to get it.

As for the problem drinker, he or she might be almost anyone you know. It might be the kid with a locker near yours in school who sneaks a drink before facing the prospect of the next class. Or the housewife who starts "nipping" some alcohol as she goes about her chores in the morning. Or the men and women who crowd into bars each evening for two or three quick ones before heading home. All of these people are more or less addicted to alcoholic beverages, even though they are still able to function on a reasonably normal level.

Besides these examples, though, there are many others where the individual's behavior gives evidence that they are no longer in control of their drinking habit. For example:

• The junior or senior high school student who manages to keep away from alcoholic beverages during the week but gets thoroughly "bombed" almost every weekend.

• The individual who manages to abstain from alcohol for months at a time, only to go off on a "lost weekend" of round-the-clock drinking until he or she reaches a point of total unconsciousness.

• The drinker who never seems to reach a state of intoxication yet can't get through a day without at least nipping every few hours.

• The teenager whose only idea of "doing something" is either to visit a bar or to buy a bottle of liquor. These people, no matter what their age, are simply looking for excuses to indulge their drinking habit.

Profile of the Problem Drinker

Obviously, within our society there are many patterns of alcohol abuse. Sometimes it takes a trained individual to recognize when a person has a true alcohol problem. In some cultural groups where liquor is socially and religiously forbidden, such as among members of the Mormon Church, any degree of drinking might be looked upon as a problem. In other groups where drinking of alcoholic beverages is common to daily life, such as the French who often drink wine with meals as frequently as others take water, it would require an almost massive amount of alcohol consumption before a person would be singled out for his excessive drinking habits. In fact, in this case the abstainer or non-drinker might be noticed for his "odd behavior" before a problem drinker is identified.

Nevertheless, most experts in the field of alcoholism agree that there are at least seven specific behavior signs which mark the problem drinker:

1. Anyone who must drink in order to function or cope with life

has a drinking problem. This would include the pre-teenage or teen-age student who needs a quick gulp of "courage" before facing a test or any other stressful situation, as well as the adult who needs a drink before calling on an important client or facing his boss. All of these people have already adopted a pattern of depending on alcohol to get them through one or more of life's daily difficulties.

2. Anyone who, by his own definition or that of the people around him or her, frequently drinks to a state of intoxication has a problem. This is the pattern of the teenager who gets "bombed" each weekend. For some reason such people cannot just take a drink socially but must imbibe until they are thoroughly drunk.

3. Anyone who goes to school or work intoxicated has a drinking problem. Some say that the man or woman, boy or girl who shows up in the morning already primed by a few drinks has reached the stage where he or she is psychologically, if not physically, dependent on alcohol. In many ways the first-thing-in-the-morning drinker is like a heroin addict who cannot function until he or she has had a "fix."

4. Anyone who habitually drives a car, operates potentially dangerous machinery, or participates in any other potentially dangerous pastime while under the influence of alcohol has a problem. Such practices indicate that the person has lost control of his or her drinking habits and is willing to accept risk—and expose those around him or her to risks—no matter what the destructive consequences.

5. Anyone who keeps bottles hidden at home, at school, at work, or in the car for quick pick-me-ups has a problem. When these people are confronted with their habit they often say, "I can stop any time I want." They rarely do, however, because they've already lost the will to go without alcohol for any period of time.

6. Anyone who drinks to the point of "blackouts," or frequently sustains some sort of injury as a result of falling while drunk, has a

problem. The same is true of people who say they can't remember where they were while drinking, what happened, or just how much they had.

7. Anyone whose drinking habits are so different from the usual patterns of alcohol consumption that they command your attention has a problem. For example, if you saw someone sitting alone at a bar, downing drink after drink, you would notice him or her because the drinking is obviously being done to blot out reality rather than as part of any social activity. By the same token, you'd notice a pre-teen drinking because any use of alcohol by children as young as eight, nine, ten, eleven and twelve is so far outside of accepted social and legal practices that it stands out. In both cases, you can only conclude that those individuals have a drinking problem.

Signs of the True Alcoholic

At what point does the problem drinker turn into an alcoholic? There is no clear line—but there are definite symptoms which indicate that a drinker no longer has any control over the habit and may, indeed, have developed a physical need for alcohol.

Alcoholism, it must be stressed, is a *sickness* in every sense of the word. Occasionally it flares up with all the drama and suddenness of an acute infection. There are cases on record of people having gone from total abstinence to chronic alcoholism in a matter of weeks. These "instant alcoholics," some scientists believe, may have some biochemical imbalance or genetic trait which makes them ultrasensitive to alcohol.

In the vast majority of cases, though, the illness builds up over a period of many years. This is one reason why experts are so concerned about the growing number of young people who are using alcohol today. Says one psychiatrist, "They are, in effect, getting a head start on the disease. The junior high student who drinks occasionally may not be dependent on alcohol today. Nevertheless, he or she is building up a tolerance to the substance and, by the time he reaches the age of twenty-five or thirty, may have a full-blown alcohol problem."

As the illness deepens, the first sign of true alcoholism may involve the morning-after miseries. The hangover that is common to even casual drinkers usually becomes a very painful episode that is marked by severe and characteristic withdrawal symptoms. These may include uncontrollable shaking or trembling, waves of anxiety, profuse sweating, hours of nausea and vomiting, and a general feeling of sickness. All of these reactions are physical signs that the body has become so accustomed to alcohol that it "cries out in anguish" when the drug is removed. Like an addict hooked on heroin, the alcoholic must have a "hair-of-the-dog" morning drink. When the alcoholic reintroduces alcohol into his or her bloodstream, the painful sensations of trembling, nausea and other morning-after symptoms are masked for another few hours.

Most alcoholics are able to hide this first stage of their disease from those around them. One teenage alcoholic, interviewed on a television talk show recently, said he'd thrown up once every morning for four years, from age twelve through sixteen, without his parents in the next room finding out about it.

How did he manage to hide his illness?

"Once I realized that I'd be getting sick each morning," he said, "I set the alarm clock for six A.M., about an hour before my parents usually got up. Then I'd go directly from my bed to the bathroom where I'd turn on the shower full force. The loud hiss of the water covered the sounds of my vomiting. I stayed there long enough to get over the first wave of sickness and then raced back to my room where

KIDS AND ALCOHOL, THE DEADLIEST DRUG

I kept a bottle hidden." This "hair-of-the-dog" usually kept him satisfied until he reached school where another bottle was hidden in his locker. And so it went throughout the day.

The second stage of the illness usually involves a complete breakdown of the drinker's moral fiber. The alcoholic may start neglecting his or her diet, health, and personal appearance in favor of an almost constant effort to get liquor and stay drunk. For most people this preoccupation with alcohol is carried on at the expense of family, friends, school attendance, marks, and reputation. And if the drinker doesn't have the financial means to satisfy his or her habit, he may take that first big step down the ladder toward skid row.

Even without the degradation of skid row, the second stage is almost certain to be marked by a worsening physical condition. This is what happened to the young man who appeared on the TV talk show. "After about two years of daily drinking," he explained to the host, "my morning-after reactions seemed to become all-day symptoms. I couldn't go for an hour between drinks without breaking out in a cold sweat, shaking uncontrollably, and getting a feeling of complete panic."

Was this what finally brought him into an alcohol treatment program? "No," he said, "it wasn't until I had my first taste of the DT's that I decided to seek help."

If an alcoholic is forced to go without liquor for a day or two, his body will quickly burn up its alcohol supply and begin to "scream" for more in the form of *delirium tremens*—"the DT's"—which produces fever, acute thirst, and hallucinations that usually take the form of terrifying voices and sights.

In the case of this teenage alcoholic, his parents finally discovered what was going on, and after carefully searching the room and removing all the hidden bottles, locked him in it. After a few days he developed his first siege of the DT's which he described as "cockroach-like bugs crawling all over the walls, ceiling, bed and onto my body."

<hr>

The Last Stages

Yet, even at this pitiful stage of alcoholism, the final slide is far from over for many people. In the most advanced stages the individual cannot function at all as a member of society. His or her energy is almost totally involved with getting drunk, staying drunk, or trying to sober up. Food becomes of such secondary importance that he becomes weaker and weaker, falling prey to malnutrition and diseases. The result is a life span that is anywhere from ten to fifteen years shorter than normal life expectancy.

Clearly, alcoholism is a vicious disease which has consequences far beyond the obvious harm to the drinker. The alcoholic is nonproductive, highly dependent, dangerous to himself and others, and extremely wasteful of our medical and social resources. Once hooked, the alcoholic can only control the habit, not cure it. Therefore, the best answer to the problem of alcoholism is to recognize the early signals and do something before they turn into actual symptoms.

5 Are You a Candidate for Alcoholism?

Everyone seems to have a theory about what makes an alcoholic. You hear, for example, that some people are born with a "genetic tendency" toward the illness. Or that it's produced by a vitamin deficiency. Or that children of heavy drinkers tend to go down the same path as their parents. Or that certain ethnic or cultural groups, such as Alaskan Indians or Irish-Americans, are particularly susceptible to alcoholism. Or that children who come from broken homes or extreme poverty situations usually turn to alcohol as a means of escape from their situation.

Would it surprise you to learn that all of these reasons are, to some extent, true? The fact of the matter is that there is no simple "model" of a typical alcoholic. Instead, there are many different kinds of drinking problems and many reasons why young people begin and continue to drink in a harmful fashion. The illness has no one cause but, rather, is the result of a variety of factors which, either singly or in combination, cause the development of problem drinking.

Perhaps this is best illustrated by the alcoholics themselves. Not long ago, I interviewed several young problem drinkers who are currently enrolled in an Alcoholics Anonymous program. Their stories demonstrated clearly that the types of people who become afflicted with alcoholism are as varied as life itself. Let's meet a few and see if you find anything familiar about them.

Patrick, we'll call him, is a seventeen-year-old who appears much younger than his actual years. Tall, frail-looking, with light-blue eyes and pale clear skin, it's hard to believe that when he walked into his first AA meeting, about a year ago, he had just come off a four-month binge of round-the-clock drinking.

"I'm the only child in a well-to-do family," he says. "I grew up with what you might call 'all the advantages.' I had my own room, my own television set, even my own telephone with a private number. In the summer, my parents sent me off to really good private camps and in the winter I went to well-known private schools. Anything I wanted, all I had to do was ask for it."

He got drunk the first time he ever tried liquor. It was at a family New Year's Eve party and there was plenty of alcohol around. "I was only five years old at the time," he recalls. "My cousin and I stole a bottle of champagne and we drank it all up in my room. He got sick and was sent to bed. But I was allowed to stay up very late, making everybody laugh with my antics. I really felt like a big deal that night."

During the next few years Patrick drank intermittently, swiping liquor from his parents' well-stocked cabinet and consuming it secretly in his room. The alcohol, he says, made him feel "important and good."

Didn't anyone get suspicious?

"Would you suspect a nine-year-old choirboy, who gets good marks in school, of being an alcoholic?" he asked.

But it was hard to hide his problem from everyone. At age ten, while attending a private parochial school in a Los Angeles suburb, he was asked to get up early one morning to help prepare the chapel for a communion ceremony. In a back room he discovered a case of sacramental wine. During the next few hours he drank three bottles and ate several bags of the holy wafers used in the Mass. The combination made him sick—"I usually could hold my liquor pretty well," he told me—and, in the middle of the communion ceremony, he vomited all over the altar. "The nuns thought I had the flu," he says, "but a priest detected the odor of alcohol and had me expelled from school."

The next few years were a succession of drinking bouts, failing performances in his classes, expulsion from schools for drinking, and increasingly painful morning-afters. His parents, now aware of the problem, shuttled him from doctor to doctor and program to program. "I kept promising to stop," he said, "but always managed to find an excuse for starting again."

Finally a psychiatrist specializing in such problems told his parents, "He's an alcoholic and won't get off the stuff until he's willing to help himself. And that probably won't come until he's touched the very bottom rung of the ladder."

That rung came one day when Patrick was convinced he was going crazy. "I'd been waking up with the shakes for weeks, tearing my room apart until I found the bottle I'd hidden," he recalled. "Once I started drinking, I couldn't stop until I passed out. Sometimes I'd get sick right in my bed, but couldn't even get up to wash or change the sheets. I'd just lie there and think, 'If I don't get out of this room I'm going to die here.'"

One morning he picked up the list of names and telephone numbers of treatment centers which his parents had placed on his desk and dialed Alcoholics Anonymous. "Come and get me," he said. "I need help." That was over twelve months ago and he hasn't touched a drop of alcohol since.

Monica's high cheekbones and slightly bronzed complexion give evidence of her half-Indian, half-Mexican background. Born and raised in a slum section of Phoenix, Arizona, she was only four years old when her father handed her a glass of wine and encouraged her to drink it. Even now, she remembers how he laughed and clapped as the warmth and excitement of the alcohol made her dance around the room.

But there were very few such happy events in her childhood. Her father deserted the family when she was seven, leaving her mother to take care of and support five children. "We lived in three rooms," she recalls, "sleeping three in a bed. Sometimes, when my mother couldn't get work as a part-time cleaning woman and the welfare check didn't come in, we lived on bread and rice for days at a time."

Occasionally, however, they did have a small windfall and then her mother would go out and buy a gallon bottle of red wine. Monica looked forward to those rare occasions because she knew there'd be a small glass at the table for her. "It always made me feel good," she says.

When Monica got to be around twelve, her dark-eyed good looks made her popular with some of the older boys in the neighborhood. "They were always drinking beer or whiskey," she explains, "and I shared their liquor because it made me part of the crowd." Soon, however, she found that she couldn't get through a day without something to drink. By age fifteen, she was a quart-a-day drinker, with most of the liquor supplied by her many boy friends. The only trouble was that she began to be sick to her stomach. One day, after retching bile and blood for almost six straight hours, she was taken to a hospital where a doctor diagnosed her condition as cirrhosis of the liver.

In adults, it usually takes about ten to fifteen years of excessive drinking to produce symptoms of cirrhosis. In children and teenagers, though, the disease often progresses at an accelerated pace, causing liver damage within a matter of months.

"Unless you stop drinking right away," the doctor told her, "you

KIDS AND ALCOHOL, THE DEADLIEST DRUG

may not make it to age twenty-one." That same day she joined an AA treatment program run by the hospital and has been alcohol-free ever since.

"As far back as I can remember," says fourteen-year-old Billy, "my parents warned me that alcohol was the drink of the devil." Instead of making him fearful of liquor, the warnings of his ultra-strict parents only served to increase his curiosity about "forbidden" substances. So when a junior high classmate offered a drink of beer, he accepted.

"Even a few swallows was enough to make me feel relaxed and free for the first time in my life," he comments. "Besides, every time I took a drink I had the idea that I was getting back at my father for the many times he punished me."

It didn't take long for Billy to become "hooked." Within a year he was drinking daily, buying a six-pack of beer on his way to school in the morning, finishing three cans even before he got to his first class and polishing off the rest before noon. Then, during lunch recess, he and another young drinker pooled their money for a bottle of wine.

When Billy drank, though, he lost all track of time and place. "Once I 'woke up' in the back seat of a city bus and the driver told me I'd been on it for hours. Another time I came to in a park about ten miles from my house." But it was when he found himself in an alley with two black eyes, his nose bloodied and two teeth—as well as his weekly allowance—missing that he decided to drop in on a treatment center. "Alcohol may not be the drink of the devil for most people," he says, "but it sure is for me."

Common Factors

It is obvious that these kids came from considerably different backgrounds and became involved with alcohol for different reasons. Yet, if we look closely at their stories we can find the "constellation of circumstances" which many researchers believe is involved in the majority of cases.

First, we can see that all of these kids reacted to their first tastes of alcohol with a feeling of intense relief and relaxation. While most people do feel "calmed" by a drink or two, the responses of these teenagers were like those produced by a powerful addictive drug. And that, in effect, is exactly what alcoholic beverages are for them.

Second, we can find in all of these youngsters some set of emotional problems which made them highly receptive to the idea of escape through alcohol.

Finally, we notice that in two of the cases, at least, there was pressure at home either to drink or to avoid alcohol at all cost. Thus the culture in which they lived produced either guilt or confusion about drinking behavior—feelings which, in turn, added to the other factors.

Does this mean that if a person doesn't fit any of these patterns he or she can drink alcohol without fear of becoming hooked? Unfortunately, the answer is *no*. Although one or more of these factors is often found in problem drinkers, scientists still don't know what causes alcoholism or how much of a role each factor plays in susceptibility to liquor. After all, there are just as many youngsters who have emotional problems or come from families where a parent is alcoholic who do not turn to liquor. "At best," says one researcher, "these factors are only leads which may help us to predict and protect alcohol-prone individuals."

Research into the Causes of Alcoholism

Although a lot of time, money, and talent has been spent trying to find out why alcoholism occurs, the state of knowledge is still very poor. Most of the theories are nothing more than ideas or unproven concepts. Nevertheless, some of the following factors, which have been observed or found in alcoholics very often, are currently undergoing scientific consideration and research:

• One avenue of research concerns people who are born with a genetic tendency toward alcoholism, just as others are born with an inborn chance of developing diabetes or hypertension. "This would explain," says one doctor, "why we see so many children of alcoholics having the same problem."

• Another approach that has come in for a lot of investigation recently is related to vitamin deficiency. It has been observed, for example, that laboratory animals which are deprived of certain vitamins will become addicted to alcohol, while others which get the vitamins manage to control their need. But these findings have not yet been duplicated in humans. And even if a vitamin deficiency were found in most problem drinkers, the scientists would then have to demonstrate whether it was the cause or the effect of drinking.

• Psychiatrists who work with alcoholics—and most work in this field is done by psychiatrically trained individuals—are aware that almost all of their patients have severe personality disorders. That is, in one way or another they are unable to cope with and adjust to life's many problems. Instead of meeting a situation head-on, they use alcohol to escape it. Once again, there is a question here of whether these emotional disorders are the cause or the result of alcoholism.

• One of the most promising avenues of study has to do with cultural and social background. There's no doubt that some ethnic or cultural groups, such as Irish-Americans, Alaskan Indians, and northern Russians, have an extremely high rate of alcoholism, while other groups, such as Italian-Americans and Orthodox Jews, have a very low rate of problem drinking. Is it environmental differences or genetic traits which account for such varying patterns? Scientists are now trying to find out.

A Formula for Avoiding Alcoholism

While the causes of alcoholism are still very hazy, the kind of environment that produces sensible drinking habits is quite clear. Generally, if you come from a culture or group where alcohol is treated in the following ways, chances are you'll handle the substance with the respect it deserves:

1. Where alcohol is consumed by adults in moderate and diluted amounts, and where children see this drinking being done within a strong family or religious setting.

2. Where the beverages used by the group are usually, though not invariably, low in alcohol content or well mixed with nonalcoholic components.

3. Where the liquor is considered more or less as a food and is almost always served in conjunction with a snack or meal.

4. Where the parents present a consistent example of moderate, controlled drinking.

5. Where alcohol is considered to be neither a virtue nor a sin.

6. Where drinking is not presented as proof of masculinity, virility, or social success.

7. Where abstinence from alcohol is not looked upon as anything unusual.

8. Where excessive drinking, intoxication, or alcohol-induced abnormal behavior is not socially acceptable. And where drinking is not considered to be stylish, comic, or a mandatory social grace.

9. Finally, and probably most important, where there are unwritten ground rules of drinking which more or less cover the above points, and where these ground rules are known and observed by most members of the culture.

6 How to Recognize, Prevent, and Treat Alcoholism

When thirteen-year-old Ginger was caught by her math teacher drinking gin out of a thermos jug which was supposed to contain chocolate milk, she received a very stern lecture. "Don't you know that liquor can do terrible things to your body?" the teacher said. "If I catch you drinking again, I'm going to send you to the principal and he'll have you expelled from school."

The teacher didn't catch Ginger drinking again—but not because she gave it up. Instead, the shy junior high student became much more careful about her drinking habits. She hid the bottles so they wouldn't be found by adults; she drank quickly and secretly in a cubicle of the girls' room; she sucked on strongly flavored mints to mask the smell of alcohol on her breath; and she adjusted her drinking patterns so she'd never show up in class or at family functions obviously drunk. Nevertheless, she did manage to consume almost a fifth of liquor a day. It wasn't until she was eighteen, in fact, that her drinking habit became so overwhelming, and the damage to her liver so massive, that she was forced to seek medical attention.

Most people still think of alcoholism as some sort of mental or moral weakness. "You've got to be strong," the math teacher told

Ginger, "and stay away from the stuff." But alcoholism is not something that can be controlled through will power. It is an illness which, in most chronic drinkers, requires medical and psychiatric treatment before it can be brought under control. The earlier this treatment is begun, the better the chances of success.

For too long, most people have thought that an alcoholic must hit "rock bottom" before he or she could be in a frame of mind either to accept or to benefit from treatment. While it is true that some individuals, such as Patrick whom we met in the previous chapter, must sink to an extremely low level before they are willing to admit they have a problem and voluntarily go in for treatment, most problem drinkers can benefit from medical help at a much earlier stage. For this reason, any sign or signal of abnormal drinking behavior should be reason enough for an individual to seek out a treatment program.

The Three Stages of Treatment

There is no simple and straightforward method of treating alcoholism. The recovery process is as complicated as the reasons why people start drinking in the first place. Moreover, the type of treatment and the stages which the alcoholic will have to go through depend on how sick he or she is when he first comes into a treatment program.

Generally, however, there are three distinct phases in most programs:

First, management of acute intoxication and the effects of withdrawal. This is essential for those "bottom rung" cases who usually seek help either during or at the tail end of a long heavy-drinking siege. As with our young friend Patrick, these people come into a treatment program while they are still "saturated" with alcohol and, oftentimes, when they are suffering from acute withdrawal symptoms.

"The initial objective in these cases," says a psychiatrist who

KIDS AND ALCOHOL, THE DEADLIEST DRUG

specializes in alcoholism, "is to rid the body completely of alcohol and its aftereffects." To do this, the alcoholic is usually put into a hospital where he or she is under constant supervision by trained professionals, and where he may even be kept under lock and key for several days. The reason for such extreme measures is to make sure he or she doesn't lay hands on any more alcohol.

During this detoxification period, the patient may receive drugs which are designed to prevent the convulsions of withdrawal, as well as medicines to increase his or her appetite and produce sound sleep. In addition, the alcoholic will be put on an extra-rich diet, possibly will receive high-potency vitamins, and most certainly will be exposed to strong emotional support from the hospital staff and doctors. All of these measures are designed to help the patient through what has been described as "that first big step back into the real world."

The second phase of most programs is the medical treatment of any health problems that may have been brought on or aggravated by chronic drinking. Most advanced alcoholics show some signs of liver disease when they are brought in; this must be halted and treated before it progresses to a point where their life is threatened. Young drinkers, too, often present some signs of secondary health problems because their tissues are particularly sensitive to the damaging effects of alcohol. In both cases, the secondary illness should be brought under control before the patient moves into a long-term program of treatment for the drinking problem.

The final phase is a treatment program designed to alter his or her long-term behavior so that the destructive drinking patterns are not continued. Sometimes such a phase will be started with a drug that discourages the patient's return to alcohol. One drug being used widely today is called disulfiram. If a patient taking disulfiram should slip and have a drink, the combination would cause violent headache, extreme nausea, and a variety of other uncomfortable symptoms. "The next time you're offered a drink," says one former alcoholic who was on disulfiram for several months, "you think twice and three times about taking it."

It should be emphasized, though, that such drugs are not designed to cure or control alcoholism. They are used only to buy time during a treatment program, until the alcoholic is ready and willing to resist liquor on his own. For long-term cure or control, the answer must come from another source.

Counseling

For the vast majority of problem drinkers, the greatest amount of benefit comes only from therapy that is designed to get at the factors which underlie or are associated with the individual's compulsive drinking habits. Several forms of therapy are available today, and what works for one patient may not do anything at all for another. Sometimes patients have to go from program to program until they find one that works in their case.

Generally speaking, the goal of all types of therapy is the same: to enable alcoholic people, young and old, to redirect their feelings, attitudes, and behavior to channel them toward more effective and rewarding patterns of living. As we've seen, most alcoholics use liquor as a means of dealing with their daily problems. Therefore, the major objective of therapy is to show the alcoholic that there are more positive methods of coping with life.

Psychotherapy

Perhaps the most widely used—and, in many cases, the most effec-

KIDS AND ALCOHOL, THE DEADLIEST DRUG

tive—form of therapy today involves an interaction between the alcoholic and a psychiatrically trained professional. This can take place in two ways.

In individual therapy, the patient has face-to-face meetings several times a week with a counselor who is either a psychiatrist or, at the least, a specially trained psychologist. The first objective of the meetings is to make the patient face up to the fact that he or she does indeed suffer from alcoholism and should not hide the problem. After that, the patient and doctor may try to find out when and how he or she uses alcohol as a "crutch." This established, they can then start to plan ways of developing and using other, healthier methods of handling problems.

Individual therapy also has the advantage of giving the patient someone he or she can trust and turn to in times of stress. This is particularly important for young alcoholics who are often lonely, full of guilt, and fearful of the world around them. The therapist becomes, in effect, the "father figure" which a youngster usually did not have in his own family. As a fifteen-year-old undergoing treatment told me, "Whenever I get the urge to take a drink, I call my doctor and we talk it out. He's a great guy."

In group therapy, which is increasingly popular these days, several alcoholics meet regularly with a trained leader. Although the group therapy method is designed to accomplish the same things as individual therapy, it has two particular advantages which are important to some alcoholics:

1. It places the alcoholic in contact with other people who share the same problem. Some patients resist individual therapy because they believe that the doctor, who isn't an alcoholic, can't possibly understand or sympathize with their plight. In group therapy, though, they have no such excuse. Moreover, the person in group therapy

can't get away with any phony reasons or rationalizations for drinking because the others have been there too and will quickly set him or her straight.

2. The group provides a means for the patient to test his or her relationship with other people, and to socialize without using the crutch of alcohol.

Involving the Entire Family

Another type of therapy that has gained wide acceptance in recent years, particularly in the treatment of pre-teens and teenagers, is family therapy. In this case the patient is brought together with his mother, father, and sometimes brothers and sisters. Under the leadership of a therapist, they gradually uncover the problems and relationships which may have either contributed to or resulted from the drinking problem. By talking about these things openly, and in a controlled environment, they help to clear the air and start the foundation of a newer, stronger, healthier family relationship.

Behavior and Aversion Therapy

Some forms of therapy are based on the assumption that alcoholism is a habit or type of behavior that can be changed through rewards or punishment. Many treatment centers which specialize in young people, for example, use behavior therapy along with other forms of psychotherapy. The teenager who stays away from alcohol for an extended period of time is rewarded for his or her "good behavior" in various ways: through added stature in the facility, better

KIDS AND ALCOHOL, THE DEADLIEST DRUG

housekeeping jobs, increased respect from fellow patients and the staff.

Aversion therapy, on the other hand, punishes the alcoholic when he or she falls off the wagon. This punishment may involve electric shock or the administration of a drug which produces a sense of suffocation and nausea any time the individual even takes a sip of alcohol. The pain and discomfort of the punishment then become associated with drinking. Hopefully, the next time alcohol is available or offered, the individual will decline.

Alcoholics Anonymous

Perhaps the oldest, best known, and most successful of all forms of treatment is the organization and technique known as Alcoholics Anonymous. AA is a voluntary fellowship of alcoholic people whose primary goal in life is to help themselves and others to get sober, stay sober, and heal the wounds that caused the drinking problem in the first place.

AA works because it places the alcoholic in an environment where everyone else shares the same problem and is dedicated to the idea of kicking the alcohol habit. As a first step, the new member must own up to the fact that he or she is an alcoholic by admitting it to the group. After that, everyone—and this may include scores of people of all ages—is ready and willing to lend support in helping the new member overcome his or her addiction. Even if the new member should get an urge to drink at three A.M., he or she can pick up a phone and call another Alcoholics Anonymous member for help. Sometimes it's only a matter of talking it out; other times it may require someone's coming over to the alcoholic's house or apartment to stay with him or her until the drinking desire passes.

Helping Families of Alcoholics

It is not only the drinkers who need help. As we mentioned earlier in this book, the family of an alcoholic also suffers and may, indeed, have very serious problems as a result of alcoholism in the family. For this reason several groups have been formed in recent years to help the nonalcoholic members of a drinker's family to understand and cope with the problems of alcoholism.

Alateen, for example, is an organization devoted to the children of alcoholics. The idea behind it is to keep pre-teens and teenagers from going down the same destructive path as their mother or father. By learning how to cope with the alcohol-related problems caused by their drinking parent, they also strengthen their own lives and gain insight into ways and means of avoiding the same pitfalls.

Al-Anon is a group set up primarily for the wives, husbands, and friends of alcoholics. Here, too, the emphasis is on explaining why alcoholism occurs, what can be done about it, and how to cope with related problems.

Where to Go for Help

When an alcoholic wants to stop drinking, he needs help quickly and efficiently. Until recently, however, it wasn't always possible to get it. In one of the nation's largest cities, for example, only one hospital bed was allocated for every 6,000 alcoholics in the area. Thus, many problem drinkers who wanted to stop often had lost their resolve by the time hospital space became available to them.

In recent years, though, the American Hospital Association has promoted a nationwide program to educate hospital personnel in the techniques of working with and treating alcoholics. "Many professionals still believe the alcoholic is a nuisance, not a sick person," says Alex McMahon, president of the American Hospital Association. "But studies by the Association show that the alcoholic is not disruptive or unmanageable or needs special facilities or time-consuming treatment." As a result, most hospitals today have facilities and trained people to work with alcoholics, and there is a new look in admitting and treating people with serious drinking problems.

Here is a small sampling of representative hospitals and the alcohol treatment facilities they offer:

Roosevelt Hospital in New York City provides both in-patient and out-patient service to alcoholics. The program is considered to be among the best in the nation. It includes both detoxification and follow-up therapy. The hospital uses a unique "scatter-bed" system which mingles alcoholics with regular medical patients. Once detoxified and pledged to stop drinking, most patients attend AA meetings.

Lutheran Hospital in Park Ridge, Illinois, has an extensive and well-equipped alcoholic rehabilitation center. In addition to working with alcoholics, the hospital has a program for their teenage children.

The Washington Center for Addictions in Boston, Mass., is dedicated solely to the problems of alcoholism and other forms of drug addiction. With over two thousand in-patients a year, the staff here has devised many techniques for working with people of different backgrounds.

Mendocino State Hospital in Talmage, California, has a large and sophisticated alcoholism center. After detoxification, the patient is given a choice of seven treatment routes which stress different areas of therapy.

St. Elizabeth's Hospital in Washington, D. C., operated by the federal government, utilizes group therapy for both long- and short-term patients.

St. Joseph's Hospital in Houston, Texas, has gained a reputation for success with "hard core" alcoholics. Various modes of psychiatric therapy are used to treat long-time drinkers.

Northwestern Hospital in Minneapolis has a twenty-eight-bed alcoholism treatment center which is designed to stimulate socializing among alcoholics.

Memorial Hospital in Long Beach, California, stresses a one-to-one relationship between patient and a recovered alcoholic on the staff. The hospital works closely with a local AA chapter.

Kings County Hospital in Brooklyn, New York, has a bold and big new program for providing alcoholism treatment to people in the poverty-stricken Bedford-Stuyvesant area.

These are just a few of the many alcoholism treatment facilities in the United States today. If you or anyone you know needs help and cannot get to one of these hospitals, then your next best move is to call your local hospital or medical society for the name and number of a treatment facility.

7 Some Questions and Answers About Alcohol

Q. Is alcoholism curable?

A. The answer really depends on your definition of the word "curable." If by curable you mean that the alcoholic, after treatment, can go back to social drinking without fear of becoming hooked again, the answer is no. Only in rare cases can an alcoholic learn to cope with his drinking problem to the point where he can continue using alcohol without fear of going on a "bender."

On the other hand, alcoholism can be controlled. This means that the problem drinker can learn how to resist the temptation of alcohol, know how to say "no, thank you" when offered a drink, and have alternate ways of coping with the personal and social problems that drove him to drink in the first place.

Q. What percentage of alcoholics actually benefit from a treatment program?

A. The percentage is very high, but not all wind up the same way or have the same amount of control. According to the National Clearinghouse for Alcohol Information, about 50 to 75 percent of all people who come in for treatment achieve a successful outcome. Although specific figures aren't available, most authorities agree that the rate of recovery for pre-teens and teenagers is probably much higher. "Regardless of the life situation," advises the National Institute on Alcohol Abuse and Alcoholism, "the earlier treatment starts after drinking troubles are recognized, the better the chances for success." This means that young people who have been drinking for only a few years have an excellent chance of controlling their habit if they enter a treatment program soon enough.

Q. Is it possible to kick the alcohol habit without entering a treatment program?

A. While it is true that a small percentage, possibly 5 to 10 percent, of true alcoholics are able to improve spontaneously, the vast majority do need the help of a medically based treatment program. For this reason you should never allow excuses such as "I can stop any time I want" or "I'll get better on my own" prevent the initiation of formal treatment.

Q. What if he or she won't go for treatment?

A. Some victims of alcoholism continue to deny their illness or reject offers of help long after they are obviously in need of professional care. In such cases, it is important to realize that entering treatment is not always a decision that depends on the attitude of the alcoholic. Concerned family members, friends and work or school associates should learn enough about the illness so they can exert firm yet compassionate pressure for treatment.

Q. How can I exert pressure without hurting the alcoholic's feelings?

A. Those close to someone who has a drinking problem should not be afraid to talk about it. So often, many of us are too polite to hurt a friend's feelings, too polite to offer help. But it isn't polite to stand by and watch a friend destroy his family and his life. Most people with a serious drinking problem really want to talk about it. Therefore, you are actually doing your friend a favor when you become involved.

Q. When is the time to get involved?

A. If you want to help an alcoholic person, you must be alert for the critical moment when he or she is most receptive to advice. Obviously, few problem drinkers will be interested in a treatment program when they are in the midst of their "high." On the other hand, almost all alcoholics will be at least receptive if they are approached while they are going through the painful experience of withdrawal and recovery from acute drunkenness.

Another critical time for offering treatment is when the problem drinker is in trouble because of his or her habit. For many junior and senior high drinkers, this could be when they are faced with the prospect of being expelled from school for their drinking habits. For others it could be when they are confronted with jail for public drunkenness or are about to lose a job.

Q. Is treatment expensive?

A. Treatment of alcoholism can range from very costly to absolutely free. Alcoholics Anonymous and the Salvation Army, for example, both offer cost-free programs. They have no dues or fees, but depend solely on voluntary contributions. Many government-supported clinics have a sliding scale of fees based on the patient's ability to pay. An increasing number of health insurance plans now provide at least some benefits for treatment of alcoholism. And most local hospitals have clinics where alcoholism is treated at moderate cost.

Q. Is there any relationship between economic class and a tendency towards alcoholism?

A. None at all! Alcoholism can strike anyone of any social or economic background. There are probably just as many alcoholics among the well-to-do as there are among the very poor. No segment of society has a corner on problem drinking.

Q. Is it necessary to abstain completely from drinking in order to avoid the pitfalls of alcoholism?

A. The decision about whether or not to drink depends on many things: religion, background, family custom, and personal preference. For some young people the choice will be clear-cut because drinking is contrary to their family and religious practices. For others, the choice will be just as evident because liquor has always been part of their family's life.

The answer, therefore, is not "to drink or not to drink," but how to live with your personal decision. And if this decision involves the use of liquor, how to do it in moderation and with control.

Q. If I decide *not* to drink, will it cause me social embarrassment?

A. There's no need to hide from the fact that you're abstaining from alcohol because your parents prefer it that way, or because you're not sure of how you'll behave while under the influence of liquor, or simply because you don't like the taste or effect of alcoholic beverages. All of these things are solid, sensible reasons for not drinking. If any of them represent the way you feel, then you should say "No, thank you" quickly, politely, and firmly. It may take guts to get the words out, but stand by your decision. Remember that you don't owe anyone an explanation for your decision, any more than they have to explain to you why they prefer to drink.

Q. Is it always illegal to serve alcoholic beverages to people under age eighteen?

A. In most states the "legal drinking age" refers to the sale or serving of alcohol in a public place. Usually—*but not always*—this does not apply to drinking in a private home or other nonpublic place. Your best bet is to find out what the local laws say about drinking, and then observe them carefully.

Q. Is being drunk in public a crime which can land you in jail?

A. Most states and municipalities today have laws on the books which make being drunk in public a crime which is punishable by a short-term jail sentence. But in some states there is a trend away from this archaic concept. In Minnesota recently, for example, the

Problem Realized?

The next step is to "ask the right questions." These questions range from, "Do you have memory lapses?" to "Do your friends think you're drinking too much?" to "Do you hide booze at home and at school?"

In many cases, the person hasn't thought of things like this because he has never been confronted with them. But once they have been pointed out, "things start to happen and they start thinking about their drinking and paying attention to it."

If a teen doesn't have a probation officer, other agencies are available for help. The Substance Abuse Group, formed by Tom Rudy and Bill Paris of the Oaklawn Center, works with teens, pointing out the alternatives to drugs and alcohol.

To become involved in this program, one can call the Oaklawn Center requesting that an appointment be set up with the group or just asking for more information.

The Logansport State Hospital in Logansport, offers a 90-day program for alcoholics. They concentrate on the education concerning alcohol, and detoxication.

Other agencies are the Northern Indiana Drug Abuse Service (NICAS) which operates out of South Bend, Booze Driars, and local Alcoholic Anonymous Centers.

However, added Mr. Miller, "The only way that we can help any teen alcoholic is if they want help in the first place, and the only way they can quit drinking is by wanting to."

Those continuing to drink may find that their jobs and school work may be affected. A Memorial teacher commented, "I haven't had too much trouble with my students drinking, but those that I have known of have had their work affected by it."

One Memorial teen added that, "I don't drink at work anymore since I got fired from two jobs for that reason. But

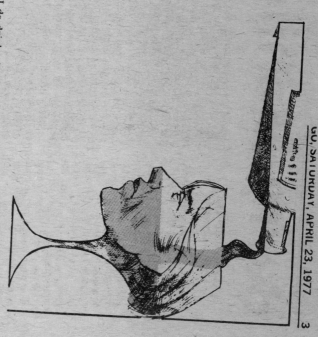

take it from there."

I do drink at school because I think lunch is about the best time to do it, and we're close to Michigan.

"Also, I don't think drinking always affects my schoolwork. If I'm worried about something at school, I drink a little and come back feeling better and able to concentrate more. But if I really drink a lot, I can't concentrate, and am not able to do my work well."

Those who do risk drinking at school may be caught and justly disciplined. In most cases, the student is expelled from school, according to Memorial counselor Dr. David Flora.

Because there is no way to determine how many teens drink alcohol, there is also no way to know how many will continue to drink. But with the help of counselors, probation officers and agencies, this number may be decreased.

In concluding, Mr. Miller commented that "all we can hope for is to plant the seed to start them thinking and let them

Drinking — More of a Than You Might Have

By LAURA SICKELS
Elkhart Memorial

Although there is no sure way of knowing the percentage, the number of teens who drink alcohol is increasing, according to probation officer Steve Miller.

Mr. Miller says that he's hearing more about teens drinking from the kids he works with. He thinks that "one reason more teens are drinking may be because they are afraid of street drugs, and the variety of things that may be in them."

A student, admitting to drinking often (about three nights a week and during lunch hour at school) remarked, "I drink because I don't like pot. It's not that I'm hooked on alcohol — it's just that I like it."

This same teen added, "You could say that drinking does help solve my problems somewhat. When I drink, I'm calmer and therefore more capable of handling my problems. The only time it would ever present a problem would be if I got caught."

While this particular teen doesn't see drinking as a problem, there is an increasing number of those who do look on drinking as a problem.

Mr. Miller thinks that "alcoholism is a disease." He also believes that "a person's chemical make-up determines whether or not he will be an alcoholic. So, real alcoholics are those who physically cannot cope with alcohol."

Many teens tend to agree with Mr. Miller who says, "one of the main reasons more teens are drinking is that it is now socially acceptable." The second most popular reason for drinking is the hope of solving one's problems.

In remembering how he first got involved with alcohol one student commented, "We were near Michigan so we went and got some beer. We got away with it and figured if we could get away with it once, we could do it anytime. So, we just kept on doing it. Now, four years later, we're still doing it.

"Usually, two or three of us go together and buy a fifth or two of Vodka or Gin. On the average, I say we each spend about $5 or $6 a week on booze," added this student.

He also stated, "I'm not ashamed of drinking, but I'm careful of who I talk to about it. I don't want my parents to

> "I drink because I don't like pot. I'm not hooked on alcohol, I just like it."

find out about it. Now, they sort of suspect something but they don't really think I'm that kind of person."

For those who think that they do have a drinking problem, and do want help, Elkhart offers agencies for this specific purpose.

First of all, a teen may receive help through the probation officer. Having worked with teens who have a drinking problem, Mr. Miller remarked that the first thing they try to do is "to make the person aware that he may have more of a problem than he thought."

"Weekend in England." His fourth and latest album, "This One's for You, on Arista, is also

ballad records may be

State Supreme Court ruled that a chronic alcoholic is not responsible for his acts and must therefore be considered as someone who is sick rather than criminal.

Q. Is alcoholism among pre-teen and teenage people found in other countries besides the United States?

A. Definitely! West German officials, for example, recently estimated that over 100,000 young people in that country, many of them between the ages of ten and twelve, were now fully addicted to alcohol. "A generation of alcoholics is growing up which will present West Germany with serious problems," Franz Vogt, a senior scientist of the Bavarian State Government, says. "There is hardly a school today where, during break periods or even during lessons, some form of alcohol is not handed around."

Similar problems are being observed in France, England, and Taiwan. Comments a Chinese physician, "What we are seeing among the young people is a reflection of what is happening to their parents."

Q. How can we prevent alcohol problems among young and old?

A. Problem drinking can never be controlled solely by treating the casualties. The ultimate goal must be prevention through early identification of the problem, the development of responsible attitudes and behavior in the use of alcoholic beverages. It also requires full respect and acceptance of an individual's choice not to drink.

References

Alcohol and Alcoholism: Problems, Programs and Progress; National Institute on Alcohol Abuse and Alcoholism, 1972.

Alcohol and Health, special report to the U.S. Congress, reprinted 1974.

Alcohol and Health: New Knowledge; U.S. Department of Health, Education and Welfare; June 1974.

Alcoholic Beverages in Clinical Medicine, by Chauncey D. Leake and Milton Silverman; Year Book Medical Publishers Inc.; 1966.

Alcoholism—a Call for Early Detection; Medical World News; October 13, 1972.

Alcoholism Held a Disease, Not a Crime; article in *AMA News*; April 21, 1969.

Alcoholism: New Victims, New Treatments; *Time Magazine*; April 22, 1974.

Juvenile Drinking, by Dr. Morris E. Chafetz; conference paper; 1973.

Like Father, Like Son, by Richard Flaste; *New York Times*; February 28, 1975.

Peer Influences on Adolescent Drinking, by C. N. Alexander and E. Q. Campbell; *Quarterly Journal of Studies on Alcohol*; 1968.

Problems of Reaching Youth, by Dr. Morris E. Chafetz; *The Journal of School Health*; 1973.

Thinking About Drinking; U.S. Department of Health, Education and Welfare; 1973.

Treating Alcoholism; U.S. Department of Health, Education and Welfare; 1974.

Young Americans: *Drinking, Driving, Dying*; U.S. Department of Transportation; 1974.

Index

abstinence, 23
abuse (alcohol), 10
accidents, 14, 26, 28
aggressive behavior, 20
Al-Anon, 52
Alaskan Indians, 37, 43
Alateen, 52
alcoholic myopathy, 27
alcoholics, 30, 33
Alcoholics Anonymous (AA), 11, 37,
    39, 41, 51, 57
alcoholism as sickness, 33
alcohol-prone, 42
American Hospital Association, 53
anesthesia, 26
aversion therapy, 50

beer, 16, 17, 18
behavior therapy, 50
"blackouts", 32
blood concentration, 25
body weight, 21
bourbon, 19
brain cells (effect on), 20, 21
brewer's wort, 18

calories, 19
cancer, 28
causes of alcoholism, 42
central nervous system, 20
Chafetz, Dr. Morris E., 14
chemistry, 17
Christianity, 16
cirrhosis, 27, 40
congeners, 22
"constellation of circumstances", 42
cost (of alcoholism), 14
counseling, 48

dehydration, 23
delirium tremens (DT's), 35
dependency (on alcohol), 32
depressant (alcohol as), 20
detoxification, 47
diet (alcohol in), 19, 28
distillation, 19
distilled spirits, 17, 18
disulfiram, 47
divorce, 14
driving, 25, 26
drop outs, 14

drug (alcohol as), 20
dumping syndrome, 22

Egyptians, 16
elementary school (alcohol users in),
    12
emotions, 26
emotional support, 47
England, 59
ethyl alcohol, 17
eyes (effect on), 25

false courage (from alcohol), 26
family, 52
family therapy, 50
Fénelon, François, 17
fermentation, 18
France, 59
fusel oils, 23

gastrointestinal ailments, 27
genetics, 33, 36, 43
gin, 17, 19
glare, 25
Greeks, 16
group therapy, 49

"hair-of-the-dog", 34, 35
hallucinations, 35
hangover, 23, 34
heart disease, 27
Hebrews, 16
heroin, 9
high-potency vitamins, 47
history (of alcohol), 16
Hunter College study, 12

individual therapy, 49
infections, 28
instant alcoholics, 33

Irish-Americans, 37, 43
Italian-Americans, 43

Kings County Hospital, 54

legal drinking age, 58
legal separation (among alcoholics),
    14
life expectancy (of alcoholics), 36
liqueurs, 17
liver disease (in alcoholism), 13, 27,
    47
long-term effects (of alcohol), 26
lost wages (caused by alcoholism), 14
LSD, 9
Lutheran Hospital, 53

malnutrition, 36
marijuana, 9
McMahon, Alex, 53
Memorial Hospital, 54
Mendocino State Hospital, 53
metabolize (alcohol), 21, 27
moral weakness, 45
Mormon Church, 31
morning-after misery, 34
motor tests, 25
murders (caused by alcoholism), 14
muscle disease, 27

National Clearinghouse for Alcohol
    Information, 55
National Institute on Alcohol Abuse &
    Alcoholism, 56
Northwestern Hospital, 54

Orthodox Jews, 43

pancreas (effect on), 28
personality disorders, 43

Phoenix House, 11
pneumonia, 28
potency, 19
pre-teens, 32, 33
problem drinkers, 29
productivity (effect on), 14
psychotherapy, 48
public drunkenness, 11

rate of absorption (of alcohol), 22
risk taking, 26
Romans, 16
Roosevelt Hospital, 53
rum, 19
rye whisky, 19

sadness (caused by drinking), 20
Salvation Army, 57
scotch whisky, 19
short-term effects (of alcohol), 25
sobering up, 23
social drinking, 26

St. Elizabeth's Hospital, 53
St. Joseph's Hospital, 54
stimulant (alcohol as), 20
suicides (caused by alcohol), 14
Synanon, 11

Taiwan, 59
therapy, 50
tolerance, 22, 34
treatment, 46
true alcoholic, 30

ulcers (caused by alcohol), 28

vitamin deficiency, 23, 36, 43
vodka, 19

Washington Center for Addictions, 53
welfare, 14
West Germany, 59
wine, 16, 17, 18
withdrawal symptoms, 34, 46

DATE DUE

30 508 JOSTEN'S